Heal Your Gut with Essential Oils

By Dr. Eric L. Zielinski

© 2016 | All Rights Reserved

Printed in the Unite States of America
First Printing, 2015

ISBN - 13: 978-0-997-16550-0

Biblical Health Publishing
2774 N. Cobb Pkwy
Suite 109-389
Kennesaw, GA 30152

www.BiblicalHealthPublishing.com

Ordering Information:

Quantity sales. Special discounts are available on quantity purchases by corporations, churches, and others. For details contact publisher at Orders@BiblicalHealthPublishing

Printed in the United States of America

Contents

Introduction

And the leaves of the trees are for the healing of the nations.

~Revelation 22:2

I can think of no other substance on earth that epitomizes this Bible verse than essential oils.

Extracted directly from the bark, flower fruit, leaves, nut, resin or root of a plant or tree, **just one drop** of an essential oil can provide the amazing health benefits that each oil provides. Used medicinally for thousands of years, the potency behind these oils is their ability to support your natural healing systems - **especially the gut!**

What we know today about the gut is opening up an entire world of limitless possibilities of how to **address the root cause** health conditions, and natural remedies like essential oils are key to helping people live free from sickness and disease. If you're looking for natural solutions to the toxic chemicals that are in your home, body and health care products then look no further. Essential oils are the answer!

~Dr. Z

How to Safely Use Oils

Pure therapeutic grade essential oils can be used safely by your family for a variety of wellness applications. However, there are several safety guidelines that you should follow when using essential oils and essential oil products.

- Remember, a little goes a long way.
- Be sure to use only pure, therapeutic-grade essential oils and follow all label warnings and instructions.
- For topical use, always dilute essential oils with a carrier oil such as fractionated coconut oil, jojoba, or almond oil.
- Essential oils should not be used in the eyes, inside the ear canal, or in open wounds. In the event of accidental contact with the eye, dilute with a carrier oil.
- Do NOT consume an essential oil internally unless labeled with a Supplement Facts box that includes specific dietary supplement, use instructions, and warnings.
- Never take more than a few drops in a gel cap, and never take more that 1 or 2 drops in water at one time.
- Discontinue the use of an essential oil if you experience severe skin, stomach, esophageal & respiratory irritation, or discomfort.
- When using on children, heavily dilute essential oils. Apply a very small amount of the oil to test skin or other sensitivity. Do not use oil on a child's hand as they may transfer to their eyes or mouth.
- Consult your physician before using essential oils if you are

pregnant or under a doctor's care, or have other safety questions regarding essential oils.

Lastly, it is important to remember that therapeutic-grade essential oils are highly-concentrated plant extracts, and should be used with reasonable care. Consulting with someone who has experience with essential oils will make your first experience with them more enjoyable and rewarding. As you learn how to use essential oils through personal experience, share your knowledge with others in a safe and responsible way and encourage others to do the same.

Healing the Gut with Essential Oils

We know that gut health can be promoted using essential oils, but what if the damage is already done?

If you are an adult in our society, chances are, this applies to you.

We've been hard on our digestive system for decades, and it's only getting worse. Not only does the food (and drink) we consume play a direct role, but lifestyle factors right down to how stressed we feel can dole out damage to the gut.

As some of the most intriguing and powerful components of herbal material, essential oils can be used as a tool to help heal the damaged gut.

Common Problems in the Gut

Sometimes, an individual's gut can be damaged without their knowledge. Perhaps the bacterial balance is off and the immune system is faltering. Maybe their emotions swing wildly, or cognitive function falters.

The gut is a command post for much of the body, with nervous system transmitters that rival the CNS in the brain and spinal cord. So even if you don't think you have gut problems – or you think you have unrelated issues – it's worth looking at your history, lifestyle, and dietary choices to consider whether you have damaged your gut in any way.

For everyone else, you know you have gut trouble because it manifests in uncomfortable, or often painful ways.

4 Gut Issues Affected by Essential Oils

Essential oils aren't always the perfect match for every gut health imbalance, but there are definite cases where their use is indicated and even preferred.

1. SIBO & Dysbiosis

The microbial balance in the gut can be shifted in many ways, usually categorized as dysbiosis. A particularly concerning form of dysbiosis is that of SIBO (Small Intestine Bacterial Overgrowth), which occurs when bacteria that should be in the colon are found in the small intestine. Both generalized dysbiosis and the more specific condition of SIBO are connected with other health concerns, including IBS and metabolic disorders. (1)Essential oils are indicated for SIBO and other gut flora issues when the essential oil is able to exhibit symptom relief without damaging beneficial bacteria. In 2012, a study analyzing the development of a probiotic (beneficial bacteria in supplement form) found certain essential oils to work well with the formula, creating a synergistic effect of increased benefits. (2)A few years before that, eight essential oils were analyzed for their effects on gut dysbiosis (bacterial imbalance). The findings included caraway, lavender, and bitter orange as stand-out examples of essential oils that would harmonize well with the beneficial bacteria in the body. (3) These studies demonstrate the excellent ability that these essential oils have to affect detrimental bacteria while remaining gentle on the body and beneficial strains. Further research for dosing and ideal treatment methods will be exciting to see!

2. IBS

Irritable Bowel Syndrome was once considered little more than a non-diagnosis – the blanket term given when doctors essentially had no idea what was going on. Now, we know that IBS not only affects more than 10% of the global population, but that fewer than 30% of those affected will ever make it to the doctor to even seek a diagnosis. (4) IBS is usually managed with diet and medication, but essential oils – especially in enteric coated capsules that can make it past the stomach – have been indicated for symptom control, as well. Although more extensive studies are welcomed, an extensive review conducted in 2008 shows peppermint oil exhibiting significant improvement over placebo, alongside dietary fiber – both of which stood alongside antispasmodic medications in efficacy. (5) To ensure the oil reaches the intestines, enteric coated capsule preparations are indicated by studies.

3. GERD

While the "gut" is technically the intestines, we usually use it interchangeably with the digestive system as a whole. As such, health trouble can start as quickly as the esophagus and acid reflux or GERD (gastroesophageal reflux disease). This combination problem is related to stomach acids (both too much and too little) as well as a faulty "flap" that should keep the acid out of the esophagus. Acid levels can be affected by lifestyle and diet, as well as bacteria. One way to approach GERD with essential oils is to use oils that protect the stomach and improve digestive processes. Ginger fits the bill, in tandem with turmeric, as indicated in a study released in January 2015. (6) The researchers tested antioxidant levels in rats with and without turmeric and ginger essential oils. The oils seemed to increase antioxidant levels as well as reduce damage done to the stomach wall. Culinary preparations would make sense here, providing a digestive system boost to your regular mealtime.

4. **Nausea**

Within the stomach, nausea is another common problem, associated with a number of ailments as a symptom ranging from unpleasant to debilitating. Anyone who has experience nausea knows that scent has a major effect on how you feel, in either a positive or negative manner. Inhaled essential oils are an excellent tool for managing nausea of nearly any cause.Backing this up with promising research, we see that peppermint and ginger work well together for alleviating nausea. (7) Refreshing citrus oils can also be beneficial, with lemon standing out as helpful for dreaded morning sickness nausea in pregnancy. (8) Aromasticks can be helpful to inhale the scent as needed, or simply open the bottle and enjoy the aroma in moments of queasiness.

Healing the Gut

We can't discuss gut health or healing remedies without discussing the importance of bacteria. Totaling more of our body composition by weight than our own cells, bacteria comprise a formidable ally or opponent, depending on the situation.
In a journal article describing the importance of gut flora, researchers detailed the "collective metabolic activity equal to a virtual organ within an organ," created by bacterial populations in the body. (9)
If you're squirming in your seat at all of this talk of bacteria, you've probably internalized the "kills 99.9% of bacteria" line that keeps us from caring about our microscopic partners in health. More likely than not, you also have gut damage to heal.

Without restoring or protecting the bacterial balance in the gut, remedies and healing techniques will be ineffective or short lived or both. Fortunately, digestive-wellness essential oils are typically safe, and will presumably be used as part of an overall shift toward holistic wellness.

Healing the Gut with Essential Oils

While these oils carry evidence of benefit to overall gut health and can facilitate gut healing, do use caution when approaching disease states. As we all know, natural products are "not intended to diagnose, treat, cure, or prevent any disease."
Essential oils are powerful and should be treated with the respect they deserve. If you have or suspect a disease or chronic ailment, seek a doctor and professional for advice.

With that out of the way, let's highlight some of the gut healing benefits of essential oils, as backed by science.

Peppermint - Like its parent plant, peppermint essential oil is known for its digestive remedy capabilities. Peppermint has long been indicated for IBS via enteric-coated capsules. (10) This was revisited in 2013, with coriander and lemon balm mentioned for their effectiveness, as well. (11)

Thyme - An antimicrobial by day, gut healer by night, thyme is a superhero in the world of gut health. For SIBO, thymol and geraniol have been shown "effective in suppressing pathogens in the small intestine, with no concern for beneficial commensal colonic bacteria in the distal gut." (12) Thymol, of course, is the major component of thyme, while geraniol is found in high concentrations in rose oil.

Lavender - Not only have we seen lavender as effective against dysbiosis, but it is a well-reputed source of anti-inflammatory and healing properties. Additionally – perhaps not coincidentally – lavender has been one of the most effective anxyolitic (anti-anxiety) essential oils, tested as a commercial internal preparation. (13) Whether the anxiety was calmed due to improved gut health or it's just a convenient double purpose, lavender is a key component of nearly any healing protocol.

Cumin - A recent study on IBS symptoms and essential oil treatments evaluated a 2% preparation of cumin essential oil in 57 patients with IBS. At the end of the four week maximum trial, symptoms including pain, bloating, and elimination problems were significantly decreased. (14)

This, of course, is just a highlight of the digestive oils. Ginger stands out for nausea and initial digestive complaints. Citrus oils are gentle and effective for both digestion and peripheral issues, like anxiety and microbial concerns. If you're serious about rebuilding your gut, essential oils should be near the top of your toolbox, researched and ready to go.

Top 8 Essential Oils for Gut Health

When we say you are what you eat, it's not just a quip or playful admonition. What enters your digestive system quite literally shapes your health. The digestive tract is a center of nutrition, of course, but also immunity and even neural processes. If the intestinal tract is faltering, the whole body suffers.

So, when we say that essential oils are good for gut health, it means they are good for whole body health, by proxy.
The tides of natural health could not have turned toward natural health at a more important time in our cultural history. Everything about our society is moving us further away from optimal gut health, shifting the balance of bacteria toward processed foods, dangerous antibiotic-resistant strains, and damaging our bodies from the inside out.

Protecting the core of our body is paramount to natural health, and essential oils are a key partner.

The Cornerstone of Wellness

Raised on the belief that microbes are inherently bad, with products that proudly claim to kill "99.9%" of bacteria, our society seems to struggle with the idea that bacteria can be – and usually are – good for you. We house bacteria on our skin and all throughout our bodies. In fact, the NIH Human Microbiome Project has proven that the human body actually contains trillions of microorganisms; literally outnumbering human cells 10 to 1! And what most people don't realize is that a major hub of microbial focus is in the gut.

It's important to understand that bacteria are most frequently our allies, because the way we approach bacteria ultimately determines how successful our attempts at wellness can be. Without beneficial bacteria to balance the deleterious strains, we are susceptible to intestinal damage, illness, mental and emotional stress, and so much more.

The Anti-bacterial Problem

Before we dive into the Top 6 Essential Oils for Gut Health, we need to address the elephant in the room: our obsession with being "clean" and killing bacteria.

There is certainly a time and a place for antibacterial effects and even antibiotics. In fact, there are essential oils that carry these actions. Sound like a contradiction? It's not. It's not the act of eliminating a bacteria that's the concern; it's the lifestyle of being antibacterial.

When we are anti-bacterial and out to destroy it haphazardly, we miss the mark in a big way.

Yet, we are interrupting healthy bacterial growth in every phase of life. Babies are increasingly born via C-section, which bypasses the mother's birth canal and loses valuable transfers of beneficial bacteria from mother to baby. (1)

In childhood, children are plastered with antibacterial hand sanitizers while parents scrub the house with antibacterial wipes and sprays – all the while killing weaker bacterial strains and allowing the more dominant to resist the component and live on.

As young adults, we often become a little to free with "junk" foods, damaging beneficial intestinal bacteria. As older adults, we've spent a lifetime damaging and otherwise eliminating bacteria, and the effects begin to surface as GERD, leaky gut, IBS, and more. Healing the gut is a topic to come, but for now let's work to overcome the struggles that we've created for ourselves in this dangerously hygienic world!

Holistic Health Solutions

With a shift in focus away from eliminating dangerous bacteria and toward strengthening good bacteria, holistic options are available to us.

Holistic refers to the body as a whole, which means we can take those first baby steps toward wellness from any area of our lives. Diet is a primary concern, improving the gut directly via the substances that come in contact with it – particularly in light of many meat sources relying on gross misuse of antibiotics that may be retained in the meat itself. (2) Cleaning supplies that do not harshly eliminate beneficial bacteria are also important, as well. Believe it or not, even stress plays a role in gut health. A Harvard educational article describes this phenomenon as the "brain-gut axis," explaining,

The enteric nervous system is sometimes referred to as a "second brain" because it relies on the same types of neurons and neurotransmitters that are found in the central nervous system (brain and spinal cord)... researchers are interested in understanding how psychological or social stress might cause digestive problems. (3)

Essential oils, if you haven't heard, can meet each of these needs – from improving the intestinal tract directly to cleaning up our cleaning products to relieving stress. If you're ready to be good to your gut, get these oils:

- Thyme & Rose
- Cardamom
- Peppermint
- Clove
- Tea Tree & Oregano
- Tarragon

Each of their preparations and actions are different, but the overarching effects spell wellness for the gut. Here are some of the best ways to use these essential oils for gut health.

Top 8 Essential Oils for Gut Health

- **Thyme & Rose** – In a study released earlier this year, researchers found that the primary constituents of thyme and rose oil – thymol and geraniol, respectively – "could be effective in suppressing pathogens in the small intestine, with no concern for beneficial commensal colonic bacteria in the distal gut." (4)
- **Cardamon** – Both anti-inflammatory and antispasmodic, cardamom is a soothing oil related to the ginger family. It has been associated with many digestive health benefits, including gastroprotective effects. (5)
- **Peppermint** – Cool and soothing, peppermint oil has been shown to improve IBS, one of the most common disruptors for gut health, when taken in a professional grade, enteric coated, commercial supplement. (6)
- **Clove** – As an oil with some of the most eugenol, clove is an efficient antimicrobial that can counter Candida albicans overgrowth. Its effects against the yeast are effective to the point that an over the counter internal preparation is being studied using clove oil. (7)

- **Tea Tree & Oregano** – A powerful duo, tea tree and oregano essential oils are the case-in-point for antibacterial as a beneficial component, compared against harsher, synthetic or toxic antibacterials. Use in DIY cleaners to help stop the spread of viral illnesses without attempting to bleach away the good with the bad.
- **Fennel** – Used as a digestive stimulant in whole-herb form, the essential oil retains some of the soothing components for the gut as an anti-spasmodic, likely connected to the estragole content. (8) This component is also found in fennel. Aromatherapy and diluted topical are very popular, but since estragole has been monitored for potential toxicity internally some recommend against ingesting it.

DIY Gut Protocol

Now that we've talked about essential oils for gut health and oils that can help to heal the gut, we can walk through ways to use them! There are dozens of oils and countless blends out there, but a few are especially beneficial for the gut, with several approaches for application and use.

When to Use Essential Oils

Essential oils are the "volatile" component of the plant, meaning they are released quickly and evaporate just as fast. This little botany tidbit can help you remember that they work especially well for quick results situations.

In other words, most essential oils are helpful for fast-acting results, such as symptom relief and antimicrobial effects.

This kind of effect matches well with gut health concerns and is amplified as part of a multipronged approach to healing the gut. Diet and lifestyle changes are imperative, and it's often worth working with a holistic healthcare professional to maximize your botanical efforts.

Taking a Whole-Body Approach

As we walk through some of the uses for essential oils and gut health, it's important to remember that you can integrate them into your whole-body approach to wellness. Suggesting an essential oils protocol or preparation does not exclude other steps toward health and healing.

For gut health in particular, essential oils pair very well with probiotics, an absolutely vital component of intestinal healing and balance. (1) They are also often used alongside digestive enzymes to maximize digestion improvement. An excellent example of early research on the combination comes with lab testing, where animals showed decreased intestinal inflammation with thymol and cinnamaldehyde essential oil components combined with the enzymes xylanase and beta-glucanase. (2)

Essential Oil Applications for the Gut

The Essential Oil Protocol for Gut Health includes evidence-based & traditional techniques to counteract concerns like nausea, GERD, IBS and more! EOs can be used in numerous ways, varying based on the oil, individual, concern, and even preference. Here are some ways to use essential oils for improved gut health.

Internal

Use capsules when you need the oil to make it to the stomach rather than the mucous membranes of the esophagus. If the oil is specifically for the intestines, enteric coated capsules are necessary, which you can find, but they can be pricey.

The important thing to remember for capsule creation is that the oils should still be diluted for extra precaution, and that the capsule shouldn't be filled with the essential oil. You still only need 2-3 drops at a time, so most of the capsule should be comprised of the carrier oil. Very small capsules are best.

Note: Internal, medicinal use of oils should be executed in proper dosing, with knowledge of contraindications and safe usage. Seek guidance or further education before creating and using capsules, or use a pre-formulated, pre-dosed essential oil supplement.

- *Optimal oils for capsule use*: peppermint, clove, ginger, oregano, tea tree, thyme. (choose 2-3 oils at a time, and mix up protocol every couple weeks).
- *Optimal situations for capsule use*: indigestion, nausea, IBS, GERD, dysbiosis, supervision by an integrative care professional
- *Carrier oil options*: coconut, almond, sesame, apricot kernel, avocado, castor, evening primrose, jojoba, sunflower, pumpkin seed, neem, hemp seed, hazelnut, borage seed.

Topical

The soothing effects of aromatherapy are translated well into massages, and an upset tummy does well with a topical application. If you keep a diluted blend or two on hand, you can quickly grab it and apply when needed.

Dilute oils to 1-3% of the total volume into a carrier oil of your choice. Favorites include coconut oil, almond oil, jojoba, and avocado oil. Do remember that if the coconut oil is exposed to temperatures below the mid-seventies, it will solidify. Fractionated coconut oil is an option if you'd like it to remain liquid and other carriers are unavailable.

- *Optimal oils for topical use*: peppermint, ginger, caraway, coriander, *fennel, anise, tarragon, thyme, citrus.
- *Optimal situations for topical use*: indigestion, constipation, stomachaches, nausea.
- *Word of Caution*: *Fennel oil (Foeniculum vulgare) contains the estrogenic compound Trans Anethole. (3) This raises obvious concerns for people with estrogen dominance and estrogen positive cancer. Also, "estragole, a main component of vulgare has become a cause of concern, as the structurally similar methyleugenol has been recently found to be a potential carcinogen. This has led to the European Union

(EU) to allow a new legal limit for estragole of 10 mg/kg in non-alcoholic beverages." (4)

Aromatherapy

Don't let a pretty scent fool you! Aromatherapy is powerful, transferring the oil's composition to your body simply by inhaling it. Inhalation is actually one of, if not the most, effective ways to administer the benefits of essential oils.

We are most familiar with diffusion, but essential oils can be inhaled much more directly for the person who is experiencing tummy trouble or gut health concerns. A couple of drops in a bowl of hot water becomes an instant personal steamer to "tent" a towel over and inhale. Jewelry or clothing can hold a drop or two for a more lasting personal source to inhale, and aromasticks can fit in pockets or purses for easy access. The simplest method? Simply open the bottle and sniff!

- *Optimal oils for inhalation*: citrus, ginger, fennel, peppermint, clove, cinnamon...or any!
- *Optimal situations for inhalation*: nausea, stomachache.

Essential Oil Digestive Blends

Now that you have a good idea of your options, you can start to connect them with overall. Blending the oils first into a carrier oil or honey will ensure proper dispersion and dilution, creating a safer and more effective remedy. For internal use, culinary or otherwise, pure, organic essential oils are ideal.

Healthy Digestion Blend
- Choose a few of the following, and blend a total of 5-7 drops into 10ml honey and carrier oil (coconut is my favorite):

clove, orange, cinnamon, rosemary, eucalyptus, lemon. Stir into tea or water, or take directly.

- Add a drop or two of the following organic essential oils as replacements in culinary preparations: ginger, fennel, dill, coriander, cardamom, cinnamon, citrus, thyme, clove, etc.

Nausea Blend

- Blend 2 drops ginger and 1 drop lemon into 5ml carrier oil. Inhale or use topically.
- Blend 2 drops peppermint and 1 drop ginger into 5ml carrier oil. Inhale or use topically.

Tummy Trouble Blend

- Choose a few of the following, and blend a total of 5-7 drops into 10ml carrier oil: thyme, rose, cardamom, peppermint, clove, tea tree, oregano, tarragon, ginger, caraway, coriander, fennel, anise. Inhale or use topically,.
- Blend one drop of peppermint in 1 tsp of honey. Add to water or tea for soothed and improved digestion, or create capsules replacing the honey with carrier oil.

A working knowledge of essential oil capabilities can be a valuable ally in times of digestive upset. Take the time to learn about each of these oils thoroughly so that you can add them to your at-home essential oil medicine cabinet and begin to heal your gut.

To help you on your journey, I have put together an Essential Oils Database on my website and have included some of the gut health-friendly oil research below.

Anise Oil

With its licorice-reminiscent flavor and scent, anise brings a refreshing and unique element to your single-oil use or combination blends. Here, we'll learn how to differentiate true anise and incorporate it into wellness routines.

Anise Plant Profile

When a common name is shared between plants, we often make the mistake of assuming they are related, similar, or even interchangeable. None of the above are necessarily true. Anise and star anise are examples, **sharing the common name of anise, but they are entirely different plants.** Latin names help us to narrow down exactly which plants we are dealing with and understand how to use them.

True anise is the plant of focus today, with the Latin name *Pimpinella anisum.* **It's part of the dill family,** a group of almost spindly annual and sometimes perennial herbs with "umbel" shaped flowering heads and strong aromatic compounds.

Star anise, on the other hand, is *Ilicium verum,* a spice derived from the pods of an evergreen tea.

Whole Herb Use

Anise seeds are usually the part of the plant used, and have been for generations. **Traditional medicine uses anise seeds** for *"carminative, aromatic, disinfectant, and galactagogue"* purposes, as well as menstrual issues, diabetes, inflammation, and more digestive issues. (1)

A good example of anise whole-herb use is found in a 2007 article in the *World Journal of Gastroenterology*. An extract of the seeds was prepared and tested on gastrointestinal health. The researchers found that it could <u>protect the gut</u> **against ulcers and lesions**, perhaps thanks to its abilities as an antioxidant. (2)

Like its relatives dill and fennel, anise is known for its <u>digestive properties</u>, particularly when the seeds are used in extracts or powders. However, there is a good deal of **essential oil content found in those seeds** that can be distilled for varying and sometimes more targeted uses.

5 Health Benefits of Anise Oil

Now that we know what anise oil is and how to use it safely, how should we use it at all? Here are three benefits and uses that are backed by research.

1. Anti-inflammatory Pain Relief

A major constituent of anise seed oil, anethole, was tested in 2014 for its pain-relieving abilities apart from simply making the individual feel sedated. The results were fairly clear that the compound helped to **lessen pain without creating sedation**, most likely thanks to anti-inflammatory actions. (3)

This backs traditional uses as a pain reliever, particularly as an oil for muscle pain and inflammatory discomfort.

Indications: Massage oil, diluted topical application.

2. Muscle Relaxant

In a similar vein, anise essential oil appears to relax muscles, which would also contribute to pain relief in many cases. To watch this action take place, researchers tested anise essential oil on pigs to evaluate the tracheal muscles' response to the application. The essential oil showed "significant relaxant effects." (4)

Not only did this study create **implications for painful, tense muscles and topical applications**, but it also demonstrated a bronchiodilatory response. In other words, breathing could improve in the case of **inflamed or congested airways**.

Indications: Topical massage of sore muscles, inhalation during respiratory illness.

3. Antifungal Options

Topical fungal infections are uncomfortable and difficult to get a handle on, and systemic yeast can be devastating. Essential oils are often effective against fungal problems, sometimes even moreso than other options. Anise in various forms, including the essential oil, seems to be **effective against multiple kinds of fungi**, including the dreaded *Candida albicans*. (5)

Indications: Diffusion, diluted topical treatments, periodic inclusion of one or two drops in a lipid dilution mixed into a full culinary recipe.

4. Antibacterial Powerhouse

Last but not least, of the anise essential oil actions we're highlighting today, antibacterial effects steal the show. Antibacterial essential oils are incredibly useful, from respiratory illnesses to skin treatments or countertop cleaning solutions.

Anise is one of the essential oils with the distinct benefit of being active against bacteria in the mouth. In one study, a decoction of the whole seed was used to demonstrate antibacterial activity. (6) The essential oil will be stronger and, diluted properly, can add to an **antimicrobial oral rinse**.

With oils that have content like estragole that require a bit of extra attention, synergy can allow you to use a little less of it while actually obtaining more benefits. **Synergy is especially important for antimicrobial benefits**, and anise demonstrates this perfectly. In a 2008 study, anise essential oil demonstrated increased antibacterial benefits when paired with thyme essential oil, one of the best-loved antimicrobials out there. (7)

5. Nausea Relief

If you think back to the last bout of nausea you struggled with, you'll remember sensitivity to smells. The right, or wrong, scent can have a bigger impact during nausea than under normal circumstances.

A 2005 study combined multiple anti-nausea essential oils – anise, fennel, Roman chamomile, and peppermint – to **create a soothing blend** for patients in hospice care. While it was not their single treatment for nausea, a majority of the patients who used the blend found improved nausea symptoms. (8) As **a non-invasive application**, we should utilize our bodies' ability to turn something as simple as a scent into a healing tool.

Indications: Personal inhalers, diffusion, on the collar of a shirt.

Anise Essential Oil Interactions

On top of the mild estragole concerns with ingestion, anise essential oil carries interactions with pharmaceutical drugs, as well. **Some common interactions** include drugs that act on the central nervous system (e.g., diazepam) and blood thinners. (9). Acetaminophen and caffeine may also change in effects when consumed alongside anise essential oil. (10)

Anise may also include phytoestrogen properties, which isn't actually a problem in most instances; **just use caution or speak with a physician** before use if you are battling an estrogenic cancer. (11)

Always discuss supplements and essential oil use with your doctor, especially if you are on medication, and **learn full interactions** before beginning to use essential oils internally. Keeping the dose to culinary levels helps to maintain safety, but drug interactions should always be a top concern.

Estragole Essential Oil Content

It's important to note that anise essential oil is a strong source of estragole, which we've discussed with fennel and tarragon essential oils as a concerning compound.

To quickly summarize, estragole itself has been flagged as a toxic compound, potentially causing cancer or creating other kinds of havoc in the body. Two **important distinctions should be made**, however, before writing off these important substances: 1) we don't consume estragole on its own, and 2) the amounts needed to replicate that risk are almost impossible to achieve. (12)

The absolute safest way to get around the controversial effects of estraagole content is to consume only the whole seed, which contains other compounds thought to mitigate the risks, or the essential oil only in very small quantities. **Pregnant and nursing women, children, and anyone with a seizure disorder** should avoid internal use to be safe.

DIY Anise Preparations

You can utilize anise for its strongest benefits in a number of ways.

- **Careful culinary inclusion** of a drop or two properly diluted in lipids and added to a recipe, remembering that less is more with essential oils

- **Antimicrobial respiratory inhalation**, combined with eucalyptus or cinnamon

- **Antimicrobial mouthwash**, with cinnamon, myrrh, and peppermint

- **Dilution into a** carrier oil for a topical muscle-relaxing massage oil

- **Whole-herb and occasional essential oil** culinary inclusion for digestive wellness

Become familiar with the safe uses of anise, as well as the GC/MS analysis from your essential oil source, which can tell you exactly how much estragole is in your anise essential oil. Then have fun experimenting with the **distinctive licorice flavor and scent** as you blend it with more familiar essential oils.

Cardamom Oil

Joining ancient aromatic spices like cinnamon and myrrh, cardamom is rich in essential oil and shares many of the benefits of these classic, fragrant substances. As a whole spice or an isolated essential oil, **cardamom is an underutilized option** for digestive wellness and antioxidant potential.

Types of Cardamom

The common name "cardamom" can refer to two entirely different plants (and their <u>essential oils</u>). *Elettaria cardamomum* is considered to be true cardamom, while *Amomum subulatum* is "greater" or "black" cardamom. Depending on where you live, you may know all of them as *cardamo<u>n</u>*, as well.

Both types of cardamom have their benefits, and if a specific type is required in the benefits in this overview, we'll note it. Still, both are from the <u>ginger</u> family, both have similar culinary benefits – though black cardamom isn't as sweet – and **both are good choices.**

Cardamom essential oils are likely to include 1,8-cineol (also found in <u>eucalyptus</u>), terpinenes, and fenchyl alcohol, among other compounds.

If you're using a cardamom essential oil for specific benefits, **make sure you know** which one your essential oil source has provided, based on the Latin name, and whether that's the oil you need.

Historical Uses

Cardamom originates in India, and as with most Indian spices, found its way to Rome in heavily utilized trade routes. (1) Through written and archaeological record, we know that **cardamom and most other traded spices were used for their fragrance** – spiritual practices, perfumery, etc. Even if the essential oil itself wasn't isolated as we are able to do today, it was still enjoyed in whatever ways they could employ.

In the Ayurvedic traditions of India, however, cardamom was used as **both a culinary spice and medicinal ingredient.** True cardamom was the variety of choice, and the fruit pods were used for digestive wellness, nausea, detoxification, oral health, and respiratory health. (2)

This was, of course, the whole or powdered spice, which does contain the essential oil in small percentages. Many of the health benefits of cardamom extend to both whole spice preparations and essential oil.

Today, as we analyze the specific compounds in essential oils and how they behave in the lab and in the body, **we are able to verify some of these actions** and apply them in our own health and wellness routines.

Top 5 Benefits of Cardamom Essential Oil

Cardamom spice as a regular dietary inclusion will mirror ancient uses, or you can utilize the more targeted benefits of the essential oil. These studies reflect some of the more **exciting things we know about cardamom** essential oil.

Some of them will be specifically about black cardamom, while most will be for the more common true cardamom. In any case, they all give us a good understanding of how best to use cardamom essential oil in our natural remedies medicine cabinet.

1. Antioxidant

As a whole spice, cardamom is among the Indian culinary choices that scavenge for free radicals and help the body to detoxify. (3) As an essential oil, black cardamom is especially potent as an antioxidant, with ***"significant activities in all antioxidant assays,"*** as well as antifungal activity. (4)

Indications: A drop in culinary preparations; topical preparations for antioxidant rejuvenation.

2. Gastroprotective

The ginger family is renowned for its digestive benefits, from healing and protective abilities to nausea relief. Like ginger, **cardamom essential oil is a good aromatherapy option for nausea**, having been evaluated for post-operative nausea with good results. (5) True cardamom in various forms, including essential oil, has been evaluated for its protective effects against ulcers, and found to have *"significantly inhibited gastric lesions."* (6)

Indications: Inhalation for nausea relief; culinary inclusion for digestive improvement and protection.

3. Chemopreventive

The potential for cancer-preventive effects of essential oils to be used in our everyday lives is exciting and promising for the future. Alongside other potent antioxidants, the **essential oil content in cardamom shows anti-tumor potential**. (7) As with all essential oils, studies are underway to determine exactly how we can best utilize these benefits to prevent cancer and perhaps treat it. Until that day, we can rest easy knowing that our regular essential oil routines are contributing to overall health.

Indications: Inhalation, topical, and culinary use to access potential chemopreventive properties.

4. Antibacterial

Essential oils of the major spices and ginger family are often antibacterial, adding a warm touch to a citrus cleaning spray. In 2007, researchers tested this group of oils for their major components and ability to mitigate the growth of bacteria. Black cardamom in particular was found to ***"inhibit growth of all tested bacteria,"* including *E. coli, Staph. aureus*, and *Listeria*.** ([8](#)) The scent of cardamom mixes well with other antibacterial oils, creating the potential for some incredible synergy in fun combinations – including antimicrobial oral rinses.

Indications: Cleaning sprays, well-diluted wound healing blends, oral health blends.

5. Antispasmodic

The category of antispasmodic covers a lot of ground: easing spasms. It can apply to digestive upsets (stomach cramps, diarrhea) and respiratory issues alike (coughing, tickle in the throat). Since we've already covered digestive wellness, we can take a look at a **traditional use of cardamom for respiratory wellness.** The presence of 1,8-cineol is our first clue, shared with the respiratory poster-oil eucalyptus. Other research has been conducted toward varying kinds of respiratory benefits, including the extract (not essential oil, but sharing some similar properties) easing symptoms of asthma. ([9](#))

Indications: Steam inhalations, personal inhalers, diffusion.

DIY Cardamom Applications

For digestive health and general wellness promotion, cardamom can be included in meal prep as a **simple addition to a healthy lifestyle**. Just blend a single drop into lipid sauces and ingredients that call for that spicy, smoky taste, before including the sauce in the full recipe. The lipid will dilute it, and the light inclusion will be both safe and beneficial.

Other applications include:

- **Antimicrobial** diffusion or sprays, with <u>citrus, frankincense, and myrrh</u>
- **Respiratory** steam inhalation, with <u>eucalyptus</u>
- **Anti-nausea** inhalation, with <u>ginger</u> and <u>peppermint</u>
- **Bonus:** include cardamom in summertime bug/mosquito sprays with lemon eucalyptus (<u>10</u>)

Ancient spices are some of the most richly scented, richly historical essential oils. Bring a touch of the past into your everyday life with the Queen of Spices, cardamom.

Cinnamon Oil

Warm, spicy, fragrant, powerful, even dangerous? What comes to mind when you think of cinnamon essential oil? Even as a potentially sensitizing oil, we shouldn't make the mistake of avoiding cinnamon altogether. There are many benefits of this classic spice and essential oil.

Cinnamon Essential Oil Sources

While we know cinnamon as simply sticks, powder, or oil, there is much more to it than a simple cinnamon source. The flavorful "sticks" we know are derived from the inner bark of a *Cinnamomum* tree, of which there are many different varieties. In fact, **cassia essential oil comes from a cinnamon tree** - *Cinnamomum cassia.*

As always, variety effects composition, and cinnamom essential oil most commonly comes from the *Cinnamomum zeylanicum* tree. From there, either the inner bark or the leaves can be harvested for distillation. This should be indicated as either "cinnamon bark" or "cinnamon leaf" on your bottle of essential oils.

And yep, you guessed it: the bark and leaf oils have their own composition, as well.

Cinnamon leaf is typically more heavily filled with eugenol – used to relieve pain and inflammation and fight bacteria – while the bark is comprised more of cinnamaldehyde and camphor –potent as an antioxidant and antidiabetic. (1)

History of Cinnamon Use

One of the oldest and most beloved spices, cinnamon was **prized in ancient times** as a costly and decadent substance, usually burned for its aroma. <u>Biblical mentions</u> include cinnamon as a "choice spice" and **part of the holy anointing oil** of Exodus.

Further east, cinnamon was used in medicinal preparations in the Ayurvedic model of medicine. It was thought to be "warming" and was used as an **antimicrobial treatment** or protective substance.

Over time, the spice trade waned and culinary preparations became standard, at least in the Western world. The ability to <u>distill essential oils</u> specifically has opened up another avenue of use for us, and **extensive research on this ancient spice** has confirmed both aromatic uses and medicinal whole-spice uses.

Top 5 Cinnamon Essential Oil Uses

Because the leaf and bark oils work differently, I'll note where one is preferred over the other. The safest use for essential oil is aromatic, via sprays and diffusion or inhalation methods. Some internal and topical use can be utilized as well, though, as long as you **carefully dilute and use appropriate amounts**. With that in mind, here are the top 5 uses for your cinnamon essential oil.

1. Antibacterial Strength

Cinnamon oil is well known as antibacterial, and that is translating to varied uses as researchers begin to think outside of the box. In 2015, a couple of interesting studies were released for uses of **cinnamon's antibacterial strength**.

The first combined antibiotic doxycycline with isolated components of 3 essential oils, one of which being cinnamon - with all three components (carvacol, eugenol, cinnamaldehyde) **found in both cinnamon leaf and bark oils**. The combination had a synergistic effect, which could imply some answers to the problem of antibiotic resistance! (2)

The second addressed an issue on our minds for awhile now, that of **oral health with natural products.** Cinnamon oil on its own was protective against an array of oral bacterial colonies. The oils didn't contain prominent levels of cinnamaldehyde, indicating a potential preference toward leaf oil. (3)

A much earlier study had confirmed more traditional uses for this antibacterial oil – **relieving bacterial respiratory conditions**. Of the essential oils tested in 2007, cinnamon and thyme rose to the top as most effective against respiratory infections. (4)

Indications: Diluted into alcohol for mouthrinse blends, cleaners, hand sanitizers, room diffusion, respiratory blends for inhalation.

2. Antidiabetic Potential

We know that cinnamon as a whole spice can be used for anti-diabetic purposes, helping to lower fasting blood sugar levels. (5) Further research is diving into the way this works, and some studies have found specific compounds of cinnamon are responsible for the effect – compounds also found in the essential oil.

For example, cinnamaldehyde in animal models has been observed **reducing glucose levels and normalizing**

responses in circulating blood. (6) In 2015, researchers found cinnamic acid to **improve glucose tolerance** and potentially stimulate insulin production. (7)

These results are promising, and it will be interesting to see how it ultimately plays out. Diabetes affects a large swath of the population, and natural remedies are needed now more than ever.

Indications: One or two drops diluted in a lipid and included in recipes; inhalation or diffusion; whole-spice culinary inclusion.

3. Antifungal Synergy

Especially with such a strong and potentially irritating essential oil like cinnamon, blending and dilution are important. Fortunately, the **oils seem to work even better that way**. A 2013 study demonstrated the effects of synergy on fungal infections, with the lavender and cinnamon blend performing the best. (8)

Incidentally, lavender sooths what cinnamon may irritate! When creating your blends, use small amounts of cinnamon to enhance the other oils in the combination for an overall effective result.

Indications: Topical fungal infections, diffusion and sprays for in-home fungal growth.

4. Gut Health Protection

Traditional medicinal uses of cinnamon essential oil include protecting the digestive system. **The whole spice is still indicated** for this purpose, but aspects of the essential oil are finding their way into studies on this topic, as well.

Eugenol, for example, found in the cinnamon leaf oil, was the subject of a study in 2000. It was found to have a **protective effect on <u>the mucosal lining</u>** against ulcers and lesions. (9) More recently, in 2015, both eugenol and cinnamaldehyde were explored as additives in animal feed for intestinal protection. (10)

Both cinnamon leaf and bark oils could be utilized here, though the leaf is much milder in taste and should contain the eugenol content that is recurring in studies.

Indications: One or two drops diluted into a lipid and added to recipes; whole-spice use in culinary preparations.

5. Cancer Fighting

Last, but certainly not least, is cinnamon essential oil's ability to fight cancer. Eighty studies to date have investigated cinnamaldehyde's ability to inhibit tumor cell proliferation via trigger cancer cell apoptosis ("programmed cell death") and other mechanisms and the research is clear: cancer patients should be encouraged that natural solutions truly do exist! (11)

Cinnamon Oil Blends and Applications

For all of its known benefits, cinnamon oil is also known as a sensitizer. The oil should always be diluted carefully, as much as a 1:200 ratio when used topically and never more than a drop or so in a full recipe. Remember that oil and water don't mix, so dilution should happen first in a lipid like coconut oil or another <u>carrier oil</u>.

Use cinnamon oil in:

- **Cleaners and sprays** with <u>clove</u> and <u>citrus</u>
- **Respiratory diffusions** with <u>eucalyptus</u> and <u>frankincense</u>
- **Culinary preparations** with sweet orange
- **Highly diluted topical treatments** with <u>ginger</u> and lavender

Dilution is the key to unlock the many benefits of cinnamon oil!

Fennel Oil

Fennel is a flowering herb hailing from the carrot family of plants. As a <u>digestive health promoting</u> **herb**, it is in good company with other beneficial herbs like dill and coriander. The seed is most commonly used in culinary preparations, though the essential oil can come from the seed or the aerial (above ground) parts of the plant.

Various preparations and applications of fennel have strong and reliable benefits, but safety is a priority with this potent essential oil.

Traditional Uses

Native to southern Europe, fennel is found in many Mediterranean recipes, much like its **closely related dill, caraway, and coriander**. Fennel's primary use in whole-herb preparations has been for digestive health. Seeds would be chewed after a meal to improve digestion, and it was included in many recipes for the same reason. (1)

While the seed was the more substantive part of the plant used, the leaves, stem, and flower are highly aromatic. Like anise, **fennel has a touch of black licorice scent** and flavor that make it uniquely suited for aromatic preparations.

While we have little evidence of fennel being used aromatically throughout history, there's no question that the ancients enjoyed the essential oil, if only as they walked by their cultivated plants and brushed the leaves, <u>releasing the oil</u>. Today, we can do far more.

4 Health Benefits of Fennel Essential Oil

Traditional uses of fennel include everything from digestive wellness to anti-inflammatory, pain relief, antioxidants, milk production, and more. The primary use would have been with the whole herb, and many believe that the concurrent compounds help deactivate the risks of estragole. (2)

The essential oil has fewer compounds, but choosing an oil that has lower estragole, using it in appropriate concentrations, and sticking to external use can help us **access the benefits of fennel** without compromising safety. Here are the top four benefits of fennel I'd like to feature.

1. Improved Digestion

Historically, fennel seeds were chewed after meals to improve digestion. More recently, fennel has been used and tested as a remedy for infant colic. It's important to note that the above concerns led to unfortunate and tragic side effects for some of the infants and the study and its methods should not be repeated.

However, we do know that *"Fennel seed oil has been shown to **reduce intestinal spasms and increase motility of the small intestine**."* (3) For adults with appropriate application, we can translate that knowledge into safe use. Including fennel in recipes and moderate internal applications, as well as including the whole seed into our diets can help maximize the digestive benefits of fennel seeds.

Indications: One drop diluted into lipids and combined into recipes; topical massage oils for stomach aches.

2. Relieved Menstrual Cramps

Fennel essential oil's antispasmodic abilities are showcased when used against menstrual cramps and dysmenorrhea. In 2001, researchers tested fennel essential oil on a rat model of menstrual issues and painful cramping. The essential oil was able to **reduce both the frequency and intensity** of some of the "cramp" contractions. (4)

The soothing actions of aromatherapy are well suited to this kind of application, as each step works together toward the ultimate goal of relief. The soothing aroma, calming effects of massage or breathing deeply, and medicinal actions work together to further the results.

Indications: Topical massage oil blended with <u>balancing herbs</u> for PMS and cramping.

3. Calmed Anxiety

A potential benefit of fennel that researchers are in the preliminary stages on is that of <u>anxiety reduction</u>. The researchers used internal applications studied on mice, finding significant and promising anti-anxiety results. (5) As an animal model, preliminary test, and internal use study, this isn't a 1:1 application to real life. However, we can utilize it in our **inhaled and topical anxiety and calming blends** to seek synergistic and added benefits. In other words: *It can't hurt to try!*

This is especially noteworthy in light of the menstrual cycle benefits just described. Both cramping and anxiety tend to be symptoms of PMS and difficult menstrual cycles, and fennel could help to relieve them.

Indications: Anti-anxiety inhalers, topical or inhaled PMS blends, diffusion during anxious times.

4. Inhibited Fungal Issues

Topical antifungals are a big over-the-counter market, yet not all are effective. Fennel essential oil provides a potential alternative, with excellent antifungal actions. From a 2015 study,

> *With better antifungal activity than the commonly used antifungal agents and less possibility of inducing drug resistance, fennel seed essential oil could be used as a potential antidermatophytic agent. (6)*

Inhibiting fungal growth in the form of athlete's foot or other topical infections, or even just in the home environment, can be difficult. This puts fennel among protective and healing sources for combating fungal issues.

Indications: Diluted into topical applications and foot soaks for antifungal treatments.

Essential Oil Composition

Fennel essential oil can be derived from the "aerial parts" (aboveground stems, leaves, and flowers) or the seeds of the *Foeniculum vulgare* plant, and the **seeds are the primary part used** in herbal and culinary preparations. Typically, the seed is what is used for essential oils, as well.

Familiar compounds like alpha-pinene and limonene are found in fennel, but the seeds contain varying – and usually high – amounts of another compound that we don't see as often: estragole. (7)

Effects of Estragole

Estragole is a phytochemical compound found in essential oils like **fennel, tarragon, and basil.** When it's part of an oil, it tends to be a *big* part of it – usually as a majority compound. Unfortunately, it's also been implicated in potential mutagenic and carcinogenic actions. This has led to much controversy, culminating in **official statements by health officials:**

> "...*Exposure to [estragole] resulting from* **consumption of herbal medicinal products (short time use in adults at recommended posology) does not pose a significant cancer risk.** *Nevertheless, further studies are needed to define both the nature and implications of the dose- response curve in rats at low levels of exposure to [estragole]. In the meantime exposure of [estragole]* **to sensitive groups such as young children, pregnant and breastfeeding women should be minimised.**" (8)

Commonsense Caution

As a fennel specific caution, one woman with epilepsy consumed an unknown amount of treats containing and unknown amount of fennel essential oil, then became unconscious for nearly an hour. (9) Safety principles derived from this information include:

- Knowing the actions, benefits, and risks of all essential oils you intend to use
- Moderating internal fennel essential oil use
- Knowing your essential oil batch's chemical profile to determine the presence of risky compounds
- Not consuming anything with an unclear label

Because of the potential risks, keeping internal use at a safe minimum and avoiding it for children and pregnant women is important. Nursing moms who know fennel to help increase milk production should choose the whole seed instead of the essential oil. By following **simple safety guidelines and commonsense practices**, we can safely enjoy the benefits of fennel essential oil.

Best Ways to Use Fennel

Fennel remains an important digestive substance in spite of safety concerns. When used in appropriate aromatherapy doses and for the appropriate circumstance, it remains beneficial. Remember:

- Pregnancy, nursing, infants and children, and seizure disorders are contraindicated
- One drop diluted into a lipid should be plenty for a full culinary recipe
- Safety is established for inhalation, topical use, and small, diluted amounts internally
- Don't exceed or override cautions without a trained and certified aromatherapist

These precautions can be considered for the other estragole-heavy essential oils, including anise and tarragon, so that you can feel confident enjoying their health and wellness benefits. Some of the best ways to use fennel include:

- **Topical antifungal treatments** with anise diluted into a carrier oil for topical treatment
- **Bath salts mixed with a topical dilution** used periodically as a foot soak
- **Topical sprays** are also beneficial for applying the treatment without leaving the skin to a moist, fungi-inviting environment

- **Relieve PMS cramping and anxiety** with a topical massage of anise and clary sage
- **Add a drop or two** of fennel to full recipes for digestive assistance

Ginger Oil

Sip some ginger ale, or have this ginger chew – it'll make your tummy feel better! I hear a mom's voice in my head when I think of the benefits of ginger. Its soothing effects on the digestive tract have been well known and beloved throughout the world for many generations.

Culinary Ginger

Ginger as we know and love it is the rhizome (part of the root) of the *Zingiber officinale* plant. At the end of the growing season, the whole plant is dug up and the rhizomes harvested for use. Some can be retained for replanting, which starts the whole process again for another year.

Ginger stores well and has a wide range of preparation possibilities, which has helped to establish it as a staple from early in human history. The harvested root can be chopped, grated, dried and powdered, even candied. It's added to both sweet and savory recipes, food and drink alike.

Traditional Uses

Not only has ginger established itself throughout history for its flavor and versatility, but its medicinal benefits are obvious and well suited to its uses. From the journal *Food and Chemical Toxicology* (linked below), ginger has been used for at least 2500 years, traditionally for gastrointestinal health, including:

- Digestive upset
- Diarrhea
- Nausea

And, in more recent years, the review notes that researchers are finding even more potential benefit, specifically in the aromatic compounds:

> *Some pungent constituents present in ginger and other zingiberaceous plants have potent antioxidant and anti-inflammatory activities, and some of them exhibit cancer preventive activity in experimental carcinogenesis.* (1)

Could ginger as digestive-aid staple have protected earlier generations from the plague of cancer that we currently face today? Details remain to be seen, but we can certainly take a page from traditional recipes to incorporate more ginger into our daily lives.

Include more ginger in your diet by making recipes such as:

- Ginger-seasoned stir fries
- Gingersnaps
- Gingerbread
- Ginger ale
- Ginger beer
- Ginger sauces
- Ginger marinades
- Ginger-seasoned desserts
- Candied ginger

The root is well established as beneficial for digestion, and you will get some amount of the essential oil compound with it, as well. For more direct benefits associated with the "pungent constituents" described above, the essential oil can be used.

Ginger Oil Composition

The essential oil is also derived from the so-called ginger root (that's actually a rhizome), via steam distillation. As with any essential oil, the actual compounds will vary based on where and how the plant is grown. Still, some of the most commonly present constituents in ginger essential oil include citral, zingiberene, and camphene, all from the terpene category of chemical compounds.

According to an analysis of ginger essential oil from a 2015 analysis, the compounds in ginger essential oil include free-radical scavenging capabilities and boosting the body's natural antioxidants. (2)

The essential oil has a spicy scent used in perfumery, inhalation, and culinary preparations.

Top 4 Health Benefits of Ginger

We love to diffuse ginger around Christmastime especially for its spicy, festive scent reminding us of holiday treats. There are some specific benefits of ginger essential oil to keep in mind when choosing oils. Ginger's benefits are primarily digestive, but you may be surprised at just how effective it might be – or what else it might be used for!

1. Gastroprotection - Ginger root has been used as a digestive aid as long as it has been used at all. Of course, the whole root carries many benefits in its various components. The essential oil itself still retains the benefit of being a digestive aid, which is both importance for potency as well as ease of use.

A recent study depicted an example of the protective effects that ginger essential oil – as well as turmeric – can have on ulcers specifically. The study was conducted in a lab on rat stomachs, but the essential oil was shown to reduce oxidative stress and reduce the damage the ulcers inflicted. (3)

Including a couple of drops of ginger essential oil in culinary preparations can quickly get it into the diet and into the stomach for a simple, easy way to pack a healing punch.

2. Nausea Relief - Probably the most reliable and definitely the easiest remedy to "apply," simply inhaling ginger essential oil is quite effective against nausea. My favorite studies on this effect is that of relief for chemotherapy-induced nausea.

A full review of the effects of aromatherapy on nausea found that, of the studies that have been conducted, *"the inhaled vapor of peppermint or ginger essential oils not only reduced the incidence and severity of nausea and vomiting." (4)* Sixty women with breast cancer volunteered to use ginger essential oils during chemotherapy, and the acute nausea as well as appetite loss and functioning were improved over placebo. (5)

Create an inhaler with some cloth that has a couple of drops of ginger essential oil, or simply open the bottle and sniff for relief of waves of nausea.

3. Inflammation - Some of the anti-inflammatory properties that no doubt aid in digestive wellness seem to also help with muscle pain. A trial using Swedish massage with ginger essential oil in short term and long term treatments found improvement in chronic low back pain, even at disability levels. ([6](#))

Add ginger essential oil to carrier oils to massage into painfully inflamed areas.

4. Cancer Prevention - Studies on cancer prevention are always exciting, and ginger joins the ranks as a potential antimutagen and chemoprotective. In other words, it could very well help to prevent cancer! Ginger essential oil performed very well against carginogens, with evidence of inhibited activity *in vitro* and the markers of their actions inhibited *in vivo* (in the body!) ([7](#))

We don't yet have indication of how to maximize these benefits, but including ginger essential oil in your regular aromatherapeutic use can only help!

Suggested Oils for Blending

Synergy is a major part of aromatherapy, which means oils typically perform better when combined with others. Try ginger with these oils for both scent combinations and effect enhancements...

- *Citrus: orange, bergamot, neroli.*
- *Floral: geranium, rose, ylang ylang.*
- *Woodsy/Earthy: eucalyptus, frankincense, sandalwood, cedarwood.*

Peppermint Oil

No, we aren't talking about mints, gum, or candy canes. Really, it's quite fascinating – in a somewhat sad way – that peppermint is so commonly associated with sweet treats rather than medicinal benefits. Aside from lavender, peppermint may be the most versatile of all of our essential oil options. And yet we've limited it to Santa Claus and toothpaste.

Considering that peppermint has the ability to:

- Treat a variety of illness from stress and migraines to skin conditions to digestive wellness
- Combat cancer cells
- Remain gentle on the skin and body
- Affect the body via respiratory, digestive, or topical applications
- Remain affordable thanks to easy propagation
- Stand up to thorough research

Is there any reason at all that we wouldn't stock our cabinets with peppermint essential oil? Our culture is seriously missing out!

History & Composition

Peppermint (*Mentha x peperita*) is a hybrid combination of watermint and spearmint that grows prolifically – in fact, it can take over like a weed. The aerial parts – flowers and leaves – are harvested for essential oil production, which is conducted via steam distillation. At this point, active ingredients typically include menthone at around 20% of the composition and menthol at roughly 40%. (1)

Typically, peppermint oil is used as an antiemetic (helps to prevent nausea) and antispasmodic (helps to prevent vomiting as well as any other harsh gastrointestinal contractions). It's a soothing digestive aid and beneficial during times of illness.

Historically, peppermint dates back as one of the oldest medicinal herbs used in Europe, an ancient remedy for both Chinese and Japanese cultures, and an Egyptian medicine in at least 1,000 B.C. When, in Greek mythology, Pluto pursued the nymph *Mentha,* he transformed her into an herb (guess which?) so that the generations to come would enjoy her just as well as he. Such a colorful legacy is contained well in this cool, accessible, effective substance.

Peppermint in the Literature

Stepping away from Greek literature and into the scientific realm, peppermint is found throughout databases of studies and reviews – even moreso when we look at its specific component *menthol.* With hundreds and literally thousands of mentions, scientists are all over this remarkable herb. I don't make promises and guarantees often, but peppermint is almost a sure thing: add it to your daily regimen and your life will never be the same.

Nausea Relief

For example, while we all hope to avoid surgery, sometimes it is a necessary part of life – and a common part of surgery is unpleasant post-operative nausea, to the tune of 1/3rd of surgical patients. In 2012, Clayton State University facilitated tests on peppermint essential oil's effects on this nasty phenomena. Moms who are in recovery from a Caesarean especially do not want to deal with vomiting and nausea on top of the mixed emotions of the joy of birth and pain of surgery, not to mention the time that could be spent bonding with their babies. So, moms were chosen for this study, with 35 respondents discovering "significantly lower" nausea levels with inhaled peppermint compared with standard treatments. (2)

Irritable Bowel Syndrome

The use of essential oils is sometimes underestimated when limited to the connotations of "aromatherapy." Topical and occasionally internal applications are relevant, as well, and one drop mixed with one teaspoon of coconut oil or (internally) honey, rubbed on the stomach or ingested, can calm an upset stomach or indigestion in a snap. This remarkable ability is being broached by researchers, marked by a systematic review of the literature that cover's irritable bowel syndrome (IBS) and peppermint.

Nine studies were reviewed, spanning more than seven hundred patients, and the conclusion was clear – taking peppermint oil in enteric-coated capsules performs much better than placebo when it comes to pain and symptom management. In their conclusion, University of Western Ontario researchers stated that, *"Peppermint oil is a safe and effective short-term treatment for IBS. Future studies should assess the long-term efficacy and safety of peppermint oil and its efficacy relative to other IBS treatments including antidepressants and antispasmodic drugs."* (3)

Bug Repellant

One of my personal favorite benefits of peppermint essential oil is bug repellant – especially since I live in mosquito country!

In a comparison of seven commercial bug repellants, Terminix® ALLCLEAR® Sidekick Mosquito Repeller nearly topped the charts. If you aren't aware, this is an "all-natural" blend that lists cinnamon, eugenol, _geranium_, peppermint, and lemongrass oils. It was very close to a tie with OFF!®, the chemical-laden, DEET-filled commercial brand. (4)

Although I don't recommend Terminix® ALLCLEAR® because I have little faith in a big name company to use true, pure, therapeutic grade essential oils, the lesson is the same. It underscores the efficiency of essential oils, no matter their quality. And an effective essential oil blend most definitely is preferred to harmful, toxic chemicals or nasty 'skeeter bites!

Top 10 Peppermint Essential Oil Uses

1. **Ease Pain Naturally**– For a natural muscle relaxer or pain reliever, peppermint essential oil is one of the best. Try using it on an aching back, toothache, or tension headache.
2. **Clear Sinuses** – Diffused or inhaled peppermint essential oil usually clears stubborn sinuses and soothes sore throats immediately. As an expectorant, the results may be long lasting and beneficial when you're down with a cold, plagued with a cough, or struggle with bronchitis, asthma, or sinusitis.
3. **Relieve Joint Pain** – Peppermint oil and lavender oil work well together as a cooling, soothing anti-inflammatory for painful joints.
4. **Cut Cravings** – Slow an out of control appetite by diffusing peppermint before meal times, helping you feel full faster. Alternatively, apply a drop or two on your sinuses or chest to keep the benefits to yourself.
5. **Energize Naturally** – Road trips, long nights studying, or any time you feel that low energy slump, peppermint oil is a refreshing, non-toxic pick-me-up to help you wake up and keep going without the toxins loaded into energy drinks.
6. **Freshen Shampoo** –A couple of drops included in your shampoo and conditioner will tingle your scalp and wake

your senses. As a bonus, peppermint's antiseptic properties can also help prevent or remove both lice and dandruff.

7 **Ease Allergies** – By relaxing the nasal passages and acting as an expectorant, peppermint can help relieve symptoms during allergy season.

8 **Relieve ADHD** – A spritz of peppermint on clothing or a touch on the nose can help to improve concentration and alertness when focus is needed.

9 **Soothe an Itch** – Cooling peppermint and soothing lavender combine again to sooth an itch from bug bites or healing sun burns.

10 **Block Ticks** – Stop ticks from burrowing with a touch of peppermint oil. Make sure you remove them by their head to lessen your chances of contracting Lyme disease!

Cautionary Common Sense

Be sure to follow professional recommendations, healthcare provider advice, and common sense when using peppermint essential oil. While it is incredible versatile and relatively gentle, it is still a medicinal-quality substance and should be treated with care. As with all oils, make sure to always dilute with a carrier oil and, as always, listen to your body and the wisdom of those who have used aromatherapy before us: essential oils are best in small doses!

Also, Harvard Medical warns that peppermint essential oil can relax the esophageal sphincter and pose risks for those with reflux. (5) Taking one or two drops of peppermint in a gel capsule can remedy this risk relatively easily. Taking one or two drops of peppermint in a gel capsule can remedy this risk relatively easily.

Tarragon Oil

Think of a fragrant dish simmering on the stove or baking in the oven – which culinary herbs and spices are you smelling? These are often full of aromatic compounds, **the essential oils escaping and making your stomach growl**. Tarragon is one such culinary herb with an essential oil element. If you haven't tried the essential oil yet, here's what you need to know.

Tarragon's Plant Profile

As a member of one of the largest flowering plant families, *Asteraceae,* tarragon is one of around 500 varieties of the species *Artemisia*. Native to Europe and Asia but thriving in North America, as well, tarragon spans traditional uses as well as modern essential oil isolation. (1)

Tarragon grows in an upright, shrub-like formation with narrow leaves and bright yellow flowers. Much like modern use, traditional preparations of tarragon varied **from culinary ingestion to medicinal extracts** and preparations. (2)

As one of the main herbs in French cooking, tarragon leaves are flavorful and fragrant. The compounds in them are understood to act as **an herbal "bitter,"** stimulating the digestive system to better process food. This can have many implications, some of which translate into the essential oil compounds.

In fact, it was the aromatic essential oil levels that garnered tarragon attention above its cousins in generations past, and it's the essential oil that stands out today.

Top 4 Tarragon Essential Oil Benefits

The whole herb is still likely the best inclusion for maximum digestive stimulation, but there are some important secondary effects that the essential oil has on <u>digestive wellness</u>, as well. Both topical and moderate internal use can yield big benefits with tarragon essential oil.

1. Antibacterial Food Safety

Often overlooked in antibacterial uses, one group of researchers took the opportunity to test **tarragon essential oil's bacteria-fighting ability** and test it in real-life application. The study, released in 2012, not only tested tarragon for its chemical properties and effects in the lab (which many studies on many products do) but also tested it in a food preservation environment.

The results told us what we already know traditionally about **essential oils: they are enhancers.** Tarragon was effective against *E. coli* and *Staph. aureus,* and was even effective in protecting cheese during the study. Confirming both aromatherapeutic traditions of blending and tarragon's contributions to food safety, they concluded:

> *Thus, it is suggested that tarragon EO be used **as a part of a combination with other preservation**...and can be applied as **a natural preservative** in food such as cheese.* (3)

In both estragole-safety and effectiveness perspectives, tarragon included as part of the overall recipe can be beneficial, enjoyable, and safe in most cases.

Indications: One to two drops blended into a lipid and added to culinary preparations, especially in combination with other culinary essential oils; cleaning blends for antibacterial surface protection.

2. Digestive Wellness

Tarragon as a whole herb carries many traditional uses for <u>digestive wellness</u>, from <u>antidiabetic</u> effects to lipid metabolism to liver protection and ulcer resistance. (4)

Translating those benefits to the essential oil isn't necessarily direct – many of the studies have centered around water infusions and alcohol extracts. As you begin to **experiment with tarragon as a culinary herb**, you can utilize a drop or two of the essential oil now and then, as well. Consider inhalation and topical belly massages, as well, to introduce digestive wellness compounds in other ways.

Indications: Use of the whole herb; some inclusion of careful internal use; blends for topical massage or inhalation.

3. Pain Relief

Often hand in hand with gastrointestinal wellness is the relief of gastrointestinal pain, and **tarragon was used to relieve both** concerns traditionally. A 2013 *in vitro* trial used an animal model to see just how tarragon essential oil might work to relieve painful conditions.

Pain relief was confirmed, validating yet another traditional use of an herb and its essential oil. (5) While the study wasn't in humans or their typical applications, the effects remain and can be utilized in whichever way is most convenient for you until we know more from direct research.

Indications: Massage oil blends, topical stomachache blends.

4. Anti-Inflammatory Swelling Reduction

The major compounds anethole and estragole found in digestive herbs like tarragon, anise, and fennel might have some controversy surrounding them, but they also carry benefits. One group of researchers evaluated the effects of anethole and estragole on swollen paws of mice. Not only did the treatment relieve the swelling, but there weren't any signs of toxicity. (6)

This doesn't tell us to throw caution to the wind, but it does demonstrate a couple of important things about tarragon and the other digestive herbs and essential oils. First, pain relief and gastrointestinal benefits are likely tied to anti-inflammatory actions. And second, toxicity in many cases depends on use. Be smart with your oils and stay safe.

Indications: Massage oil and other topical blends, especially for swelling, sore muscles, and inflammatory illness.

Estragole's Controversial Twist

Before we get into the ways you can use tarragon essential oil, it's important to know what you cannot do. One of the main components of the essential oil content in tarragon is called *estragole*, which can also be indicated as *methyl chavicol* and *chavicol,* among other names. (7)

Reviewing similar cautions for fennel essential oil, you'll find that **many whole herbs known for their digestive prowess also have concentrated estragole** in their essential oils. The complexities of nature are so intriguing!

The bottom line for estragole safety is to use your essential oil in absolute moderation and wisdom. Ask your supplier for a copy of the GC/MS evaluation to **know how much estragole is in that batch** of tarragon, and only use it internally if the percentage is low and the dilution high. Russian tarragon, for example tends to be low in estragole. In preparations, one or two drops for an entire meal is more than enough to suffice.

Official safety statements for estragole confirm that moderation is key – toxicity levels were far above anything we'd actually consume – however, a few demographics should minimize use (8):

- **Pregnant or nursing women,**

- **Children, and**

- **Individuals with seizure disorders.**

With that said, tarragon has stood the test of time, and it seems the essential oil will, as well. Here are some of the reason's tarragon (used safely) isn't going away.

How to Use Tarragon

As more research is conducted, we will undoubtedly learn details that will improve our use. Learning how essential oils like tarragon work in the body, why estragole is concentrated in digestive herbs yet not without its controversial effects, and **the best ways to get the most out of an oil** will come to light bit by bit, study by study. For now, we can mimic traditional wisdom in light of what we do know. Some suggested tarragon uses include:

- **Stomachache** topical blend, including oils like lavender

- **Culinary** essential oil use, with one or two drops per recipe and partner oils like <u>sweet orange</u>

- **Topical** treatments for antioxidant skin health

- **Massage oil** inclusion for easing tense, painful muscles

- **Whole-herb** use, taking advantage of the entire composition of tarragon to mitigate estragole and allow for fewer safety concerns

Conclusion

The thief comes to steal, kill and destroy. I have came that they may life and have it abundantly!

~ John 10:10

I hope you have enjoyed this journey down the road of learning how essentials oils can help heal your gut and how they can affect your entire body. If you haven't tried them yourself, I strongly encourage you to give them a try. You won't be disappointed if you give your medicine cabinet a makeover!

Essential oils are a wonderful way to take charge of your own health and learn about natural solutions and remedies to everyday problems. Keep on digging and you'll find the answer to unlocking your Abundant Life health potential in no time!

Shalom!
~Dr. Z

References

Healing the Gut with Essential Oils

1. http://www.ncbi.nlm.nih.gov/pmc/articles/PMC3099351/
2. http://www.hindawi.com/journals/grp/2012/457150/
3. http://www.ncbi.nlm.nih.gov/pubmed/20030464
4. http://www.ncbi.nlm.nih.gov/pmc/articles/PMC3921083/
5. http://www.ncbi.nlm.nih.gov/pmc/articles/PMC2583392/
6. http://www.ncbi.nlm.nih.gov/pubmed/24756059
7. http://www.ncbi.nlm.nih.gov/pubmed/22784340
8. http://www.ncbi.nlm.nih.gov/pubmed/22784340
9. http://www.ncbi.nlm.nih.gov/pmc/articles/PMC1500832/
10. http://www.ncbi.nlm.nih.gov/pubmed/9430014
11. http://www.ncbi.nlm.nih.gov/pubmed/24283351
12. http://www.ncbi.nlm.nih.gov/pubmed/25500493
13. http://www.ncbi.nlm.nih.gov/pubmed/26293583
14. http://www.ncbi.nlm.nih.gov/pmc/articles/PMC3990147/

Top 8 Essential Oils for Gut Health

1. http://jn.nutrition.org/content/138/9/1796S.full
2. http://www.nytimes.com/2013/03/28/opinion/antibiotics-and-the-meat-we-eat.html?_r=2
3. http://www.health.harvard.edu/newsletter_article/stress-and-the-sensitive-gut
4. http://www.ncbi.nlm.nih.gov/pubmed/25500493
5. http://www.ncbi.nlm.nih.gov/pubmed/16298093
6. http://www.ncbi.nlm.nih.gov/pubmed/9430014
7. http://www.ncbi.nlm.nih.gov/pubmed/26170621
8. http://www.ncbi.nlm.nih.gov/pubmed/26434144

DIY Gut Protocol

1. http://www.hindawi.com/journals/grp/2012/457150/
2. http://www.ncbi.nlm.nih.gov/pubmed/25275341
3. http://www.ncbi.nlm.nih.gov/pubmed/12818366

Essential Oil Profile: Anise

1. http://www.ncbi.nlm.nih.gov/pmc/articles/PMC3405664/
2. http://www.ncbi.nlm.nih.gov/pubmed/17373749
3. http://www.ncbi.nlm.nih.gov/pubmed/25506382
4. http://www.ncbi.nlm.nih.gov/pubmed/11137352/
5. http://www.ncbi.nlm.nih.gov/pubmed/16375827
6. http://www.ncbi.nlm.nih.gov/pubmed/16935829
7. http://www.ncbi.nlm.nih.gov/pubmed/18226481
8. http://www.sciencedirect.com/science/article/pii/S0962456205000706
9. http://www.ncbi.nlm.nih.gov/pubmed/22926042
10. http://www.ncbi.nlm.nih.gov/pubmed/26619825
11. http://www.ncbi.nlm.nih.gov/pubmed/13680814
12. http://www.ema.europa.eu/docs/en_GB/document_library/Scientific_guideline/2010/04/WC500089960.pdf

Essential Oil Profile: Cardamom

1. http://www.ncbi.nlm.nih.gov/pubmed/25278182
2. http://www.allayurveda.com/elaichi-herb.asp
3. http://www.ncbi.nlm.nih.gov/pubmed/18997285
4. https://www.researchgate.net/publication/233685960
5. http://www.ncbi.nlm.nih.gov/pubmed/22392970
6. http://www.ncbi.nlm.nih.gov/pubmed/16298093
7. http://www.ncbi.nlm.nih.gov/pubmed/23886174
8. http://www.ncbi.nlm.nih.gov/pubmed/17960105
9. http://www.banglajol.info/index.php/BJP/article/view/8133

10.   http://www.ncbi.nlm.nih.gov/pubmed/22242564

Essential Oil Profile: Cinnamon

1.   http://www.ncbi.nlm.nih.gov/pubmed/21929331
2.   http://www.ncbi.nlm.nih.gov/pubmed/26631640
3.   http://www.ncbi.nlm.nih.gov/pubmed/26165725
4.   http://www.ncbi.nlm.nih.gov/pubmed/17326042
5.   http://www.ncbi.nlm.nih.gov/pubmed/21480806
6.   http://www.ncbi.nlm.nih.gov/pubmed/17140783
7.   http://www.ncbi.nlm.nih.gov/pubmed/25765836
8.   http://www.hindawi.com/journals/ecam/2013/852049/
9.   http://www.ncbi.nlm.nih.gov/pubmed/10930724
10. http://www.ncbi.nlm.nih.gov/pubmed/25553481
11. http://www.ncbi.nlm.nih.gov/pubmed/?term=cinnamaldehyde+cancer

Essential Oil Profile: Fennel

1.   http://www.sciencedirect.com/science/article/pii/S1878535212000792
2.   http://www.ncbi.nlm.nih.gov/pubmed/22899959
3.   http://www.ncbi.nlm.nih.gov/pubmed/12868253
4.   http://www.ncbi.nlm.nih.gov/pubmed/11448553
5.   http://www.ncbi.nlm.nih.gov/pubmed/25149087
6.   http://www.ncbi.nlm.nih.gov/pubmed/25351709
7.   http://www.ncbi.nlm.nih.gov/pubmed/20334152
8.   http://www.ema.europa.eu/docs/en_GB/document_library/
     Scientific_guideline/2010/04/WC500089960.pdf
9.   http://www.ncbi.nlm.nih.gov/pubmed/21865126

Essential Oil Profile: Ginger

1.   http://www.ncbi.nlm.nih.gov/pubmed/17175086
2.   http://www.ncbi.nlm.nih.gov/pubmed/26197557
3.   http://www.ncbi.nlm.nih.gov/pubmed/24756059

4.   http://www.ncbi.nlm.nih.gov/pubmed/22784340
5.   http://www.ncbi.nlm.nih.gov/pubmed/26051575
6.   http://www.ncbi.nlm.nih.gov/pubmed/24559813
7.   http://www.ncbi.nlm.nih.gov/pubmed/24023002

Essential Oil Profile: Peppermint

1.   http://www.ncbi.nlm.nih.gov/pubmed/19768994
2.   http://www.ncbi.nlm.nih.gov/pubmed/22034523
3.   http://www.ncbi.nlm.nih.gov/pubmed/24100754
4.   http://www.ncbi.nlm.nih.gov/pubmed/23092689
5.   http://www.health.harvard.edu/staying-healthy/
        understanding_and_treating_an_irritable_bowel

Essential Oil Profile: Tarragon

1.   http://www.academicjournals.org/article/article1390551311_Tak%20et
        %20al.pdf
2.   http://link.springer.com/article/10.1007/s11094-008-0064-3
3.   http://www.ncbi.nlm.nih.gov/pmc/articles/PMC3391558/
4.   http://discovery.ucl.ac.uk/1352036/1/Obolskiy-et-al2011-Art-
        dracunculusJAFC%5B1%5D.pdf
5.   http://www.ncbi.nlm.nih.gov/pubmed/24074293
6.   http://www.if-pan.krakow.pl/pjp/pdf/2012/4_984.pdf
7.   http://webbook.nist.gov/cgi/cbook.cgi?
        ID=C140670&Mask=4&Type=ANTOINE&Plot=on
8.   http://www.ema.europa.eu/docs/en_GB/document_library/
        Scientific_guideline/2010/04/WC500089960.pdf

About the Author

Founder of DrEricZ.com, **Dr. Eric Zielinski** is a sought-after Biblical Health educator, author and motivational speaker. Inspired by the timeless principles in the Bible, Dr. Z's mission is to provide people with simple, evidenced-based tools that they need to experience the Abundant Life. By creating programs like Beat Cancer God's Way and hosting online events such as the Essential Oils Revolution and the Heal Your Gut Summit, Dr. Z educates people in natural remedies and empowering life strategies. He lives in Atlanta with his wife and three children.

Dr. Z Around the Web:

https://www.facebook.com/drericz
http://www.pinterest.com/drericz/
https://twitter.com/DrEricZielinski
https://instagram.com/drericz/

74310774R00040

Made in the USA
Middletown, DE
22 May 2018